Keto Diet Miracle in 7-Steps, Instantly Lose Weight Now and Discover a New You

Ironclad Ketogenic Diet System to Take Back Your Life with a Meal Plan Included

Dr. Michelle Danville

Disclaimer:

© 2017 – TWK - Publishing. All Rights Reserved.

No part of this publication may be reproduced, stored or transmitted in any form or by any means – electronic, mechanical, scanning, photocopying, recording or otherwise, without prior written permission from the author.

This publication is provided for informational and educational purposes only and cannot be used as a substitute for expert medical advice. The information contained herein does not take into account an individual reader's health or medical history.

Hence, it's important to consult with a health care professional before starting any regimen mentioned herein. Though all possible efforts have been made in the preparation of this e-Book, the author makes no warranties as to the accuracy or completeness of its contents.

The readers understand that they can follow the information, guidelines and ideas mentioned in this e-Book at their own risk. All trademarks mentioned are the property of their respective owners.

Table of Contents

Introduction

I want to thank you and congratulate you for downloading *Keto Diet Miracle in 7-Steps Instantly Lose Weight Now and Discover a New You.*

So far, I have already tried a dozen diet plans and most of them were recommended by famous personalities of our time. At first, my purpose was to simply lose weight and get my slim figure back until an unimaginable event occurred in my life. It made me realized that I really should lose weight and to seriously consider nutritious and healthy meals and not just follow some diet fad.

I did some research and found out that I can be slim and healthy at the same time. All of the diet fad that I tried left me weak and irritated most of the time. I often starve and always end up cheating – not a good example to follow. Among the different (healthy) diet plans that I've read, ketogenic diet made my curiosity rise to an unbelievable level. Eat more healthy fats to lose weight and be healthy? I mean, come on! Anyone who tried different types of diet fad should know better than that, right?

I read on and did more research on ketogenic diet and understood everything. I admit that I was still a bit apprehensive to try it (after spending so much time reading all of those stuff) but I still did. It was not easy at first, but I got the hang of it. I was keen on losing weight while keeping a healthy body. I have set my mind that I really need to do it and I am glad I did.

Today, I can walk the streets with confidence and I feel light. I have never felt this way in years and the best thing about it is that I know I have a healthy and fit body. That's why I have decided to share my good fortune to all of you through this book. I hope you too can look and feel better than you ever did before.

This book contains the important, life-changing 7 steps that you need to take towards a new you. It provides essential information about ketogenic diet that can help you claim your life back. This book will:

- Help you understand what keto diet is.

- Guide you on how to start with ketogenic diet.

- Teach you the different food that can help you achieve ketosis, lose weight, and gain better health.

- Explain how you can attain your goal and keep a healthy and fit body for life.

- Enumerate different quality fats and how to incorporate them in your diet.

- Discuss the importance of protein in ketosis.

- Furnish other important information that can help you reach your objectives without so much fuss.

It is important to set your goal before you start planning and remember to set a realistic one that will make you work hard to achieve it. Setting a goal that is too high may frustrate you when you don't reach it. Setting a goal that can be easily achieved is also not advisable because you won't get a lot of benefits.

The Ketogenic diet can bring amazing things to you. As a precautionary measure, it is recommended to seek your physician's opinion first before you try any diet program.

Thanks again for downloading this book, I hope you enjoy it!

Chapter 1
Understanding the Keto Diet

The primary purpose of ketogenic diet was to help children with epilepsy and make them respond efficiently to anti-epileptic medications, which should be taken regularly. A ketogenic diet usually consists of large portion of fats, small portion of carbohydrates, and adequate portion of protein.

The Ketogenic diet got its name from its ability to mimic the effect of fasting in order to produce ketones. Due to the absence of carbohydrates to burn during fasting period, the body has no other option but to use fats for fuel. The main source of energy in a ketogenic diet is fat and when you combine this with small portion of carbohydrates, your body will generate ketones.

Once the food you ate turned into glucose, it will be distributed to the cells in your body to be used as energy source. Glucose is also the brain's typical source of energy. When there's only too little carbohydrates to convert into glucose, your liver will process fats to provide energy (in the form of ketone bodies and fatty acids) to the brain. Ketosis happens when your body uses fat, instead of carbohydrates, to turn into fuel. Several studies have shown that seizure reduction has something to do with keto diet, which children with difficult to manage epilepsy were advised to consume.

Let us take a look at ketogenic diet's history to understand it better.

Brief History of Ketogenic Diet

For hundreds of years, medical practitioners tried to treat epilepsy using different dietary remedies. Among the tried dietary remedies, fasting showed the most promising result. One doctor hinted that the effects of fasting could also be achieved with the right diet – more particularly, the ketogenic diet.

Hundreds of years ago, people believed that epilepsy was associated with evil spirits. The disease piqued the interest of Hippocrates, the legendary Greek physician. He openly declared that epilepsy was not caused by evil spirit but something biological. It was

Hippocrates who made use of fasting as a means to counter the disease.

Records revealed that Hippocrates was not the only one who used fasting to combat the disease. There were other physicians who mentioned fasting as an effective alternative to stop epilepsy from manifesting.

In the early part of the 20th century, fasting (as a means to treat epilepsy) attracted the interest of people all over the world. Its popularity elevated even more when two doctors from Paris, named Marie and Guelpa, helped minimize the effects of epilepsy on 20 people. They even documented the entire process and presented it in their report.

Soon after, doctors that belonged to different medical fields in the United States drew the same conclusion when they used fasting to improve the condition of their patients. However, fasting was just a great temporary cure.

Transition to Ketogenic Diet

William Lennox of the Harvard Medical School was able to establish a connection between fasting and ketogenic diet. Later, he made the transition from fasting to keto diet.

During his observation, he learned that seizures began to recede after fasting for two to three days. He arrived at the conclusion that the condition got better due to metabolic change – to be more precise, a change in the body's energy source.

Lennox suggested that the body began burning fat for fuel when the primary energy source was unavailable. The discovery made by Lennox was paramount in the ketogenic diet development.

In 1921, Dr. Rollin Woodyatt discovered the presence of beta-hydroxybutyric and acetone in people who had undergone a fast or followed a diet that was high in fats and low in carbohydrates. Beta-hydroxybutyric and acetone belong to ketone family. Dr. Woodyatt's discovery created a massive impact on Dr. Russell Wilder who also made an amazing discovery that year.

Dr. Wilder recognized that fasting was effective but unsustainable. The good doctor explained that the same ketone bodies that were generated during fasting can also be produced when a patient eats a kind of diet (ketogenic to be precise) regularly. Dr.

Wilder named the diet as ketogenic due to prolonged state of ketonemia.

Dr. Peterman of Mayo Clinic has standardized the diet that Dr. Wilder discovered. He presented these calculations:

- 10 to 15 grams of carbohydrates each day

- 1 gram of protein for every kilogram of bodyweight

- The remaining portion for calories must be filled with fat

The given proportions are basically the same with today's diet save for some minor alterations.

Using Dr. Peterman's metrics as guide, other doctors started experimenting with the new diet that was a blessing for patients with epilepsy. Dr. Peterman also noted the wonderful effects of ketogenic on the brain of a patient with epilepsy.

The ketogenic diet became the best weapon against epilepsy. It was so effective in hindering effects of epilepsy that it became the pharmaceutical industry's topmost rival in 1938, the year when the first antiepileptic drugs were introduced.

The next three decades were gloomy for ketogenic diet when antiepileptic drugs overshadowed it. Most patients with epilepsy chose the drugs because they offered a better option than keto diet – patients with epilepsy no longer need to follow a strict diet just to keep their epilepsy under control. However, there were still those who continued with the diet.

Another oil diet was developed in 1971. Its aim was to entice people to give diet another shot, but it proved to be futile. So many years passed by and the ketogenic diet was seldom mentioned and antiepileptic drugs became even more popular. The drugs enjoyed the limelight for so many years until an episode of Dateline was aired in 1994 about a boy named Charlie Abrahams.

For the first two years, Charlie suffered from what seemed to be endless seizures. His parents tried everything from faith healing to brain surgery. They tried everything, except giving Charlie a ketogenic diet.

While searching for epilepsy treatment, Charlie's father Jim Abrahams discovered the ketogenic diet. They immediately took Charlie to John Hopkins where he started his keto diet. It did not take long before they saw favorable results. Charlie was able to control his seizures and showed significant cognitive development, which his doctor thought was unlikely to happen. Jim was puzzled because no one mentioned about ketogenic diet earlier. No one informed them regarding the wonderful things it can do for children with epilepsy.

Charlie's case was able to bring back the prestige that ketogenic diet was able to enjoy during its earlier years. Today, medical practitioners recommend keto diet for a number of reasons including weight loss.

What is Ketosis?

Ketosis is a natural metabolic process wherein fats get burned for energy. Our body usually burns carbohydrates for fuel. A ketogenic diet has a large portion of fats and only meager portion of carbohydrates. When your body has no carbohydrates to burn for energy, it will naturally use the stored fats. Such action will result in build-up of ketones.

There are people who encourage ketosis by adhering to the ketogenic diet. The purpose of said diet is to make the body burn the stored or unwanted fats. It compels the body to depend on fat as its source of energy. When you follow a ketogenic diet, you will be able to lose weight.

Due to limited carbohydrates that can be turned into glucose as energy, your body has no other option but burn fats to generate fuel. It would be impossible for you to function well if you have no energy to get you going. When you do a lot of activities, your body will naturally burn more fats (in the absence of carbohydrates) to provide continuous flow of energy. You will definitely lose weight when you burn so much fat.

Important Things to Remember About Ketosis

There are few important things that you need to remember about ketosis and they are:

- Ketosis happens when the body fails to gain sufficient access to glucose, which is its main source of energy.

- Ketosis is a condition where the stored fats are broken down to generate energy, which also produces a type of acid known as ketones.

- The acidity of blood increases as ketone levels get higher. It could cause ketoacidosis, which is a serious condition that can lead to death. It has the ability to alter the normal functioning of the internal organs like the kidneys and liver.

- Individuals who have type 1 diabetes have higher possibility to develop ketoacidosis. An emergency medical treatment is necessary to prevent or give remedy to diabetic coma.

- Some people who would like to lose weight turn to ketogenic diet to force their body to burn stored fats instead of carbohydrates.

Apart from losing weight and epilepsy, the ketogenic diet could also help improve the following conditions:

- Metabolic syndrome

- Diabetes

- Cardiovascular disease

- Levels of HDL (high-density lipoproteins, the "good" cholesterol)

However, it is not advisable to follow a ketogenic diet for a long period of time.

Experts are also conducting some studies regarding the possible beneficial effects of ketogenic diet on the following:

- Lou Gehrig's disease

- Polycystic Ovary Syndrome (PCOS)

- Cancer

- Acne

- Alzheimer's disease

Keto is not recommended for everyone. You should not try ketogenic diet if you are (any of the following):

1. Suffering from autoimmune conditions or serious health issues.

2. Currently on medication for diabetes.

3. Taking medication for high blood pressure or hypertension.

4. Pregnant or currently breastfeeding.

5. Being too skeptical about it (you need to consult your doctor to clear your doubts; it

could be that you already feel that there's something wrong with your body).

Step 1 to a New You – State Your Weight Loss Goal

You must clearly state your weight loss goal and do everything in your power to achieve it. You can set up a goal that is:

Specific – point out the exact weight that you want to lose.

Measurable – make sure that you will be able to measure your goal (in this case, you can use a scale to help you out).

Attainable – your weight loss goal must be realistic and possible to achieve. It is fine to set a rather ambitious goal but make sure that you have the means and capabilities to achieve it.

Relevant – a relevant goal means it is something that truly matters to you and your decision is not being influenced by someone else. Your weight loss goal must not create conflict with your other goals in life.

Time bound – you need to set a specific time frame to reach your goal and make sure that you do.

Once you have set your weight loss goal, it is wise to have an accountability partner that can help you check or track your progress. Your accountability partner is your weight loss or fitness buddy that can make you stick to your weight loss plan.

Choose an accountability partner that you can trust and someone who is willing to help you achieve your goal. That person should be someone who won't accept your lame excuses for defying your own weight loss plan. It is best if you can find someone who has a schedule that's compatible with yours. In case it's not possible, you can check on each other by sending messages. Doing so will remind you regarding the weight loss goals you both set for yourselves.

Here is a list of accountability partner that you may want to consider:

- family member (including relatives)

- significant other (spouse or partner)

- close friend

- counselor

- colleague

- member of your church

- member of your club or organization

- support group

- social media friend

There are also sites that offer their services to be your accountability partner and you need to pay a certain fee.

You've only just begun. You still have 6 more steps to go. Make sure to see it through the end so you can meet the new you.

Chapter 2
Getting Started with Keto Diet

It is advisable to plan ahead if you want to start a keto diet. You can calculate how fast you can get your body into a ketogenic state by watching what you eat. The more you restrict your carb intake (consuming 15 grams or less per day), the faster you will enter ketosis.

Know your Current Status and Where You Intend to Be

Being overweight can lead to serious health issues and other unfavorable outcome. If you want to attain a slim, fit, and healthy body, you need to know the current status of your body first. It can help you gain a better understanding on where you want to go in terms of weight loss.

To know your current fitness, you can go to this BMI calculator. You also need to consult your doctor to perform other health assessments. It is best to know your current health status to make sure that it is safe for you to follow a keto diet.

If you want to manually compute your BMI, you can use this formula:

$$BMI = \frac{\text{weight in kg.}}{\text{height (in meters)}^2}$$

If your BMI is:

- less than 18.5, you are underweight

- between 18.5 and 24.9, you have healthy or normal weight

- between 25 and 29.9, you are overweight

- 30 or higher, you are already considered obese

Keep in mind that when you follow a keto diet, your meal must always be high in fats, has a moderate amount of protein, and low in carbohydrates. Typically, you can consume 20 to 30 grams of net carbs in your daily diet. However, keeping your glucose levels and carbs intake low can bring better results. If you want to follow a keto diet to lose weight, it is best to watch your total carbs and net carbs.

Basically, the ratio of macronutrients has the following ranges:

- 5% to 10% of calories from carbohydrates

- 15% to 30% of calories from protein

- 60% to 75% (or more) of calories from fat

After determining the right ratio for carbohydrates and protein, you can fill the remaining portion with healthy fats. If you have an active body, you may need to add more protein but don't make it bigger than the portion allotted for fat.

You can go to this keto diet calculator to know your ideal macronutrient intake that can help you achieve a slim and fit body. Your body fat and body weight will surely change when you strictly follow the keto diet. You need to recalculate your macronutrients every month so you will know the most ideal intake that can help you achieve your weight loss goal.

You only need to weigh yourself once a week. There are times when you won't be able to see any difference in your weight – this is still considered normal. Women may experience fluctuations in weight more often than men. There are fluctuations that have something to do with hormonal imbalance and water retention.

Step 2 to a New You – Minimize your Carb Consumption

It is not that easy to make a transition to the ketogenic diet. You can start minimizing your carb consumption first. It is better if you can include high quality oils in your diet, such as MCT (medium-chain triglyceride) and coconut.

MCT Oil and your Diet

Medium-chain triglyceride is a type of saturated fatty acid that offers a lot of benefits. One of the great sources of MCT is coconut oil. Only 62 to 65 percent of coconut oil's fatty acids are medium-chain triglycerides. Recently, concentrated MCT oils are becoming more popular.

Standard Western diets are lacking in MCTs. It may be due to the fact that people have always believed that all saturated fats can bring harm to the body. However, there were studies that showed that dietary saturated fat has nothing to do with increased risk of cardiovascular disease (CVD) or coronary heart disease (CHD).

Ideally, MCT oils or coconut oil must be included in your daily diet. Certain saturated fats, like MCTs and coconut oil, are easier to digest than LCTs (long-chain triglycerides) that include nuts, soybean oil, olive oil, and more.

MCTs can be digested fast and get absorbed by the liver. Once MCT gets to your liver, it creates a thermogenic effect and can alter your metabolism in a good way. This is one of the reasons why a number of people state that MCTs are quickly burned by the body for fuel and won't add to your fat storage.

Other good sources of MCT include palm oil as well as grass-fed butter, whole milk, full-fat yogurt, and cheese.

Coconut Oil and your Diet

Coconut oil has a large amount of naturally occurring MCT oil, which can also be found in butter and palm oil. There's a huge difference between coconut oil and most dietary fats. Most food contain long-chain fatty acids, while coconut oil consists mainly of medium-chain fatty acids. Between long-chain and medium-chain, the latter metabolizes quickly and goes directly to the liver after passing through the digestive tract. They can be turned into ketone bodies or be used immediately for fuel. No part of it goes to the fat storage.

Several studies on Pacific Island people, who typically get their calories (30 to 60 percent) from coconut oil, have all shown almost zero rate of cardiovascular disease. In a study, a group of rats was fed with long-chain fats and another group was fed with medium-chain fats. The rats that consumed medium-chain fats had 23% less body fat and 20% less weight. When you click this link you will be redirected to over 1,500 studies that can prove the many health benefits of coconut oil.

This oil has many uses and health benefits. It can help your body absorbs magnesium and calcium better. It can help speed up your weight loss when you include it in your meals. It can also make you sleep better.

There are also studies that show it can help enhance insulin levels.

Coconut Oil vs. MCT Oil

The main difference between coconut oil and MCT oil is that the latter is more concentrated and contains different MCTs while coconut oil contains lauric acid and medium-chain triglyceride. MCT oil contains only MCTs and nothing else.

Medium-chain triglyceride has four different types. They differ according to the number of carbons attached to fat molecules. Coconut oil contains only one type of MCT called lauric acid. The body can turn lauric acid into monolaurin, which has anti-protozoa, anti-bacterial, and anti-viral properties. Even so, most people prefer concentrated MCT oil because it usually contains all types of MCTs that are hard to obtain from other food.

Coconut oil has naturally occurring MCT, while some concentrated MCT oils must be processed in a laboratory to contain all types of medium-chain triglyceride.

Given the differences, coconut oil and MCT oils proved to be beneficial and a great addition to your keto diet. It is best to start adding these two oils in your diet as part of your good fats because they can be used immediately for energy and won't add to your fat storage.

Chapter 3
Diet and Nutrition

Avoid consuming refined carbs such as fruit, starch (beans, potatoes, legumes, etc.), or wheat (cereals, pasta, bread, and similar foods). However, you can consume berries, star fruit, and avocado in moderation.

To get the net carbs, use this formula:

$$\text{Net Carbs} = \text{Total Carbs} - \text{Fiber}$$

Foods You Can Eat Freely

Let this list be your guide when preparing your keto diet.

Wild Animal and Grass-Fed Sources

These are rich in omega 3 fatty acids known to be heart-friendly. You need to stay away from meat and sausages that are wrapped in breadcrumbs. It is also best to avoid meat and hotdogs with starchy or sugary sauces.

1. Pastured eggs

2. Gelatin

3. Grass-fed butter

4. Offal

5. Ghee

6. Wild-caught fish & seafood (avoid farmed fish)

7. Pastured pork and poultry

8. Grass-fed meat – venison, goat, beef, and lamb

9. Grass-fed organ meats – kidneys, heart, liver, and others

Healthy Fats

You need to include lots of healthy fats in your keto diet.

1. Saturated

2. Polyunsaturated (PUFA)

3. Monounsaturated (MUFA)

Non-Starchy Vegetables and Fruits

1. Summer squash – zucchini, spaghetti squash

2. Cucumber

3. Asparagus

4. Bamboo shoots

5. Celery stalk

6. Leafy greens – spinach, radicchio, chives, Swiss chard, lettuce, bok choy, and endive

7. Some cruciferous vegetables – radishes, kohlrabi, and kale with dark leaves

8. Avocado

Natural Sweeteners

If you have a sweet tooth and simply can't part from sweet things, you can use the following:

1. Stevia

2. Monk Fruit

3. Inulin

4. Erythritol

5. Swerve

It is still best to start training yourself in eliminating sweets in your life to stop your craving.

Beverages and Condiments

It is best to make homemade condiments and beverages to make sure that there are no additives that can harm your body.

1. Water

2. Tea – black, herbal, and others

3. Coffee – black, with coconut milk, or with cream

4. Pickles

5. Homemade bone broth

6. Mustard

7. Pesto

8. Mayonnaise

9. Fermented foods – sauerkraut, kombucha, kimchi, and others

10. Crushed crackling or pork rinds for breading

11. All herbs and spices

12, Lime or lemon juice plus zest

13. Whey protein without additives, soy lecithin, hormones, and artificial sweeteners

14. Egg white protein

Food You Can Only Eat Occasionally

There are types of meats, vegetables, and fruits that are best to eat occasionally.

Vegetables and Fruits

1. Some cruciferous vegetables – rutabaga, turnips, fennel, Brussels sprouts, broccoli, cauliflower, red cabbage, green cabbage, and white cabbage

2. Nightshades – peppers, tomatoes, and eggplant

3. Berries – mulberries, cranberries, strawberries, blueberries, raspberries, blackberries, etc.

4. Sea vegetables – kombu and nori

5. Okra

6. Globe or French artichokes

7. Sugar snap peas

8. Water chestnuts

9. Wax beans

10. Leek

11. Bean sprouts

12. Parsley root

13. Rhubarb

14. Winter squash (pumpkin)

15. Mushrooms

16. Garlic

17. Coconut

18. Spring onion

19. Olives

20. Onion

Grain-fed Animal Sources

You are also allowed to eat grain-fed meat only if grass-fed meat is not possible to obtain at such time. You are only allowed to eat a limited number of grain-fed meats. As much as possible, always choose grass-fed meat. You should avoid consuming farmed pork at all costs because it contains high amounts of omega-6 fatty acids, which could lead to fatty acids imbalance that may yield negative effects.

1. Beef

2. Eggs

3. Poultry

4. Ghee

5. Bacon

Full-Fat Dairy

You need to avoid low-fat products because they usually contain sugar and starch and can only provide meager sating effect.

1. Cheese

2. Sour cream

3. Cottage cheese

4. Full-fat yogurt

Nuts and Seeds

1. Sunflower seeds

2. Sesame seeds

3. Pumpkin seeds

4. Macadamia nuts

5. Flaxseed

6. Pine nuts

7. Hemp seeds

8. Hazelnuts

9. Walnuts

10. Almonds

11. Pecans

12. Brazil nuts (eat in moderation due to very high level of selenium)

Fermented Soy Products

Make sure to consume only non-GMO (genetically modified organism) and fermented soy products.

1. Paleo-friendly coconut aminos

2. Soy sauce

3. Tempeh

4. Natto

5. Unprocessed black soybeans

6. Green soy beans or edamame

Condiments

Those who prefer to consume paleo-friendly fares should bear in mind that xanthan gum is not paleo-friendly. However, there are some paleo diet enthusiasts that only need a measly amount. Choose extra dark chocolate between 70% and 90% and watch out for soy lecithin. You also need to be careful of sugar-free mints and chewing gums because they may contain carbs.

1. Sugar-free tomato products - ketchup, passata, puree

2. Healthy sweeteners – Stevia, Erythritol, Swerve, and others

3. Thickeners – xanthan gum and arrowroot powder

4. Cocoa powder

5. Carob powder

6. Extra dark chocolate

Fruit, Vegetables, Fruits, Seeds and Nuts with Average Carbohydrates

There are some fruits, vegetables, seeds, and nuts that contain small amounts of carbohydrates that you can still eat occasionally. Don't develop a habit of consuming them every now and then. It is still best if you avoid them.

1. Root vegetables – sweet potato, parsnip, beetroot, carrot, and celery root

2. Watermelon

3. Honeydew

4. Galia

5. Cantaloupe

6. Chestnuts

7. Cashew nuts

8. Pistachio

9. Fresh figs

10. Pears

11. Kiwifruit

12. Dragon fruit

13. Cherries

14. Kiwi berries

15. Nectarine

16. Plums

17. Orange

18. Grapefruit

19. Apple

20. Peach

21. Apricot

Alcohol

Drinking alcohol occasionally is fine if you only want to maintain your weight. However, you need to completely avoid drinking alcohol if you are trying to lose weight.

1. Unsweetened spirits

2. Dry wine

3. Dry red wine

Food that You Must Avoid Completely

The foods that you need to avoid completely are genetically modified, rich in carbohydrates, and/or full of preservatives.

1.   All grains – sprouted grains, quinoa, buckwheat, barley, rice, rye, amaranth, sorghum, millet, corn, bulgur, oats, and wheat

2. White potatoes

3. All grain products – crackers, cookies, bread, pasta, etc.

4. Sugar and sweets – soft-drinks, sweet puddings, ice creams, high-fructose corn syrup, agave syrup, and table sugar

5. Artificial sweeteners – sweeteners that have Aspartame, Saccharin, Sucralose, Acesulfame, Equal, Splenda, etc.

6. Zero-carb, low-carb, or low-fat products – diet drinks and soda, gluten, mints and chewing gums, etc.

7. Processed food that contain carrageenan like products using almond milk

8. Products that contain monosodium glutamate

9. Products that contain sulphites

10. Wheat gluten

11. Products that use BPA (Bisphenol A) packaging materials

12. Tropical fruits – papaya, banana, mango, pineapple, etc.

13. High-carb fruit – grapes, tangerine, etc.

14. Fruit juices (all-natural and processed)

15. Dried fruits in large quantities – raisins, dates, etc.

16. Refined fats or oils – corn oil, grape seed oil, soybean, canola, cottonseed, safflower, and sunflower oil.

17. Trans fats – margarine, hydrogenated vegetable oil, etc.

18. Farmed fish

19. Factory-farmed pork

20. Milk (you are only allowed to consume raw, full-fat milk in small amounts)

21. Sweet, alcoholic drinks – cocktails, sweet wine, beer, etc.

Now that you have the list of foods that you are allowed and not allowed to eat, you should be able to plan your keto diet with ease.

Step 3 to a New You – Plan your Meal (Week Long Plan Included)

You plan your meal according to your macronutrients number (use the keto diet calculator in Chapter 2). For starters, you can repeat the same breakfast, lunch, or dinner that you had the previous days for an entire month or two as you try to gather more keto recipes.

Let us start with easy and simple keto meal plan sample that can serve as your guide.

Day 1

Breakfast: Berries and Nuts with Creamed Coconut Milk

Fat   : 56.5 grams
Protein   : 11.2 grams
Net Carbs   : 9.8 grams
Calories   : 584

1/2 cup creamed coconut milk

30 grams almonds

1/8 teaspoon cinnamon

1/4 berries (choose from the approved list)

Get a bowl and combine all the ingredients well. Serve and enjoy.

Lunch: Keto-Friendly Tuna Salad

Fat   : 49.8 grams
Protein   : 59.7 grams
Net Carbs   : 3.9 grams
Calories   : 713

2 tablespoons mayo

2 pieces hard-boiled pastured eggs, sliced

Splash of lemon juice

1 small head lettuce, shredded

1 medium spring onion, coarsely chopped

1 6.3-ounce can tuna in brine, drained and flaked

Salt to taste

Get a bowl and combine all ingredients. Mix well and serve.

Dinner: Egg Muffin and Green Salad

Fat   : 38.3 grams
Protein   : 18.2 grams
Net Carbs   : 4.6 grams
Calories   : 454

Ingredients for Egg Muffin:

2 large pastured eggs

1/2 cup frozen spinach

Salt to taste

Get 2 ramekins and put half of the ingredients in each dish, and microwave for 1 to 2 minutes. You can also choose to add smoked salmon, pastured bacon, pastured ham (check your macronutrients for the right proportions). Set aside.

Ingredients for Green Salad:

1/2 avocado

2 cups crispy greens, coarsely chopped or torn

Salt to taste

1 tablespoon olive oil

Some lemon juice

Put all the ingredients in a bowl and toss well to combine.

Get your egg muffin and serve it together with the salad. Enjoy.

Dessert: Squares of Lindt 90%

Fat	: 9 grams
Protein	: 3 grams
Net Carbs	: 3 grams
Calories	: 105

You only need 2 squares of Lindt 90% for your dessert.

Day 2

Breakfast: Keto Style Omelet

Fat   : 47.3 grams
Protein   : 38.7 grams
Net Carbs   : 2.1 grams
Calories   : 608

1 tablespoon ghee

3 large pastured eggs

100 grams left-over slow-cooked meat, shredded or sliced

Salt to taste

Beat eggs in a bowl and season with salt. Heat the pan, add ghee, and pour in egg when oil is hot enough. Transfer into a plate and add meat on top. Fold and serve with half cup Sauerkraut.

Lunch: Easy Salad

Fat   : 38.2 grams

Protein	: 15.5 grams
Net Carbs	: 5.2 grams
Calories	: 441

2 hard-boiled pastured eggs, sliced

Splash of lemon juice

1 small head lettuce, coarsely shredded

Half avocado, sliced

1 medium spring onion, coarsely chopped

1 tablespoon extra virgin olive oil

Salt to taste

Combine everything in a bowl and toss well. Serve and enjoy.

Dinner: Chops and Asparagus

Fat	: 43.7 grams
Protein	: 35.2 grams
Net Carbs	: 4 grams
Calories	: 566

2 tablespoons ghee or lard

1 medium pork chop

1 large bunch of asparagus, hard part removed

Some lemon juice

Salt to taste

Season your pork chop with salt and set aside. Season the asparagus with salt and splash some lemon juice. Heat pan over medium heat and add 1 tablespoon ghee. Pan-roast your meat and put it on a plate when cooked. Use the remaining ghee to pan-roast your asparagus. Put it on a plate and serve together with your pork chop.

Dessert: Coco-Choco Cups

This recipe makes 20 Coco-Choco Cups, and each cup has the following nutrition information:

Fat   : 25 grams

Protein   : 2 grams

Net Carbs   : 1 gram

Calories   : 240

Ingredients for candy cups:

3 tablespoons powdered Swerve

1/2 cup shredded coconut (unsweetened)

1/2 coconut oil

1/2 coconut butter

Ingredients for topping:

3 ounces dark chocolate (sugar-free), melted

Prepare a mini-muffin pan with 20 holes or two mini-muffin pans with 10 holes each. Put mini-muffin liners in each hole. Put a small saucepan over low heat. Add in coconut oil and coconut butter. Stir until melted and combined. Add in shredded coconut and stir for a bit. Add sweetener to combine well. Take out from heat and let it cool for a bit. Stir once in a while. Pour equal amount of mixture in each muffin hole. Freeze for about 30 minutes or until firm to the touch. Spoon the melted chocolate on each muffin cup and wait for it to set before you can serve. You can keep the candies for a week.

Breakfast: Wild Salmon and Egg

Fat   : 25.4 grams
Protein   : 30.9 grams
Net Carbs   : 8.7 grams
Calories   : 421

1 tablespoon ghee

1 large pastured egg

1 cup braised spinach

1 cup blackberries

1 package wild salmon, smoked

Salt to taste

Fry egg in ghee and transfer to a plate. Neatly arrange the smoked salmon and spinach on the plate with fried egg. Season with salt and serve with blackberries.

Lunch: Green Salad and Roasted Prawns

Fat   : 45.8 grams
Protein   : 30.9 grams
Net Carbs   : 1.9 grams
Calories   : 564

2 tablespoons extra virgin oil

1/4 cup black olives, pitted and sliced

2 cups fresh chard, coarsely shredded

200 grams uncooked prawns

1 tablespoon ghee

Cayenne pepper and salt to taste

Put pan over medium heat and add ghee. Season the prawns with cayenne pepper and salt before you put them in the pan to roast. Get a large bowl and combine all the untouched ingredients. Mix well. Add seasoning if needed. Serve roasted prawns with green salad and enjoy.

Dinner: Lettuce Wrap and Tomato Salad

Fat   : 34.7 grams
Protein   : 30.5 grams
Net Carbs   : 8 grams
Calories   : 479

Ingredients for Lettuce Wrap:

1 small head lettuce

150 grams left-over meat, sliced or shredded

Wrap some meat in lettuce leaf, secure it, and place on a plate. Do the same with the rest of meat. Set aside.

Ingredients for Tomato Salad:

1 tablespoon extra virgin olive oil

1 tablespoon fresh basil, chopped

1 medium spring onion, sliced

1 cup cherry tomatoes, quartered

Salt to taste

Combine all ingredients and toss well. Serve salad together with the wrapped meat.

Dessert: Keto Macaroons

This recipe makes 10 macaroons, and each has the following nutrition information:

Fat	: 5 grams
Protein	: 1.8 grams
Net Carbs	: 0.5 grams
Calories	: 46

3 egg whites

2 tablespoons Swerve

1 tablespoon coconut oil

1 tablespoon vanilla extract

1/2 cup coconut, shredded

1/4 cup almond flour, choose organic

Put a medium bowl in the freezer to chill. Mix Swerve, coconut, and almond flour in a bowl until well combined. Put a small saucepan over medium heat and add coconut oil. Add vanilla extract next. Add coconut oil mixture to the flour mixture. Blend well. Take out the chilled bowl and put in egg whites. Whisk until you get stiff peaks. Gently fold the egg whites into the flour mixture. Be careful not to over mix, you need to preserve the foaminess of egg whites.

Prepare a baking sheet and divide the mixture into 10 equal parts. Arrange them on the baking sheet and bake for 8 minutes at 400°F. Take it out of the oven if you see a nice golden brown color on top.

Breakfast: Berries and Nuts with Creamed Coconut Milk

(See Day 1 for macronutrient details and recipe)

Lunch: Taco Salad

Fat	: 42 grams
Protein	: 36 grams
Net Carbs	: 12 grams
Calories	: 570

1/4 cup sour cream

1/4 avocado

3 ounces ground beef

1.5 ounces cheddar cheese, grated

3 pieces cherry tomato, sliced or quartered

2 cups lettuce, chopped

2 teaspoons taco seasoning

Salt to taste (optional)

Prepare a skillet over medium heat and brown the beef. Add taco seasoning and some salt. Set aside. Put some meat in your plate and add slices of cherry tomato and avocado as well as lettuce, sour cream, and grated cheese. Enjoy.

Get another heaping until you finished everything. You can also choose to mix everything in one go, although it may not look as appetizing as doing it a little at a time.

Dinner: Green Beans and Roasted Salmon

Fat   : 42.2 grams
Protein   : 46.5 grams
Net Carbs   : 8.9 grams
Calories   : 1,670

200 grams green beans

2 tablespoons ghee

200 grams salmon fillet

Salt to taste

Some lemon juice

Season the fish fillet with salt and a splash of lemon juice. Put a pan over medium heat and add 1 tablespoon ghee. Add in salmon and cook until tender. Transfer in a plate. Stir-fry green beans using the remaining ghee. Add the cooked green beans in the plate that contains roasted salmon. Serve and enjoy.

Dessert: Choco Fat Bombs with Macadamia

This recipe makes 6 bars, and each bar has the following nutrition information:

Fat	: 28 grams
Protein	: 3 grams
Net Carbs	: 3 grams
Calories	: 267

1/4 cup coconut oil

4 ounces macadamia, chopped

2 tablespoons Swerve

2 tablespoons cocoa powder, unsweetened

2 ounces cocoa butter

Melt cocoa butter in a double boiler. Add cocoa and mix well. Put in Swerve and stir until well blended. Add chopped macadamia, stir, and add coconut oil. Blend well and turn off heat. Prepare 6 square molds and put in square paper cups. Pour mixture into the molds and make sure to distribute evenly. Let it cool for a while and refrigerate to harden.

Day 5

Breakfast: Avocado, bacon and eggs.

Fat: 54.4 grams

Protein: 22.5 grams

Net Carbs: 3.8 grams

Calories: 623

1 tablespoon ghee

2 thick slices of bacon

2 large pastured eggs, beaten

1 small spring onion, chopped

Half avocado, sliced

Salt to taste

Heat pan over medium heat and add ghee. Add spring onions and some salt to the beaten eggs. Add egg mixture to the pan and scramble. Transfer to a plate and set aside. Fry bacon and set it together with the scrambled egg. Add avocado and serve.

Lunch: Green Salad and Roasted Prawns

(See Day 3 for macronutrient details and recipe)

Dinner: Egg Muffin and Green Salad

(See Day 1 for macronutrient details and recipe)

Dessert: Creamy Vanilla Pudding

This recipe makes 4 servings, and each has the following nutrition information:

Fat   : 37.5 grams

Protein   : 8 grams

Net Carbs   : 7.8 grams

Calories   : 399

90 grams walnuts, chopped

170 grams fresh berries of choice

10 drops Stevia (liquid form)

1 teaspoon alcohol-free vanilla extract

1 can coconut milk (full fat), chilled

Mix vanilla, Stevia, and coconut milk in a bowl. Whisk until well combined. You can use an electric mixer and whip for 30 seconds. Get another bowl, add in walnuts and berries, and mix well. Set aside. Prepare 4 jars and divide the cream pudding into 4 equal parts. Divide the walnuts mixture into 4 equal parts. Fill each jar with alternating layers of cream pudding and walnut mixture. Top with some ground cinnamon.

Breakfast: Scrambled Eggs, Mushroom, and Ham

Fat   : 37.8 grams
Protein   : 28.2 grams
Net Carbs   : 5.8 grams
Calories   : 490

1 tablespoon ghee

1 thick slice ham, coarsely chopped

3 large pastured eggs, beaten

Bunch of chives, chopped

1/4 cup cherry tomatoes, sliced

1 large portobello mushroom, stem and gills removed

Olive oil

Preheat oven to 390°F. Put the portobello on a baking sheet, brush it with olive oil, and bake for 12 minutes. When it's done, take it out and set aside. Add ghee in a pan, put in chopped ham and stir for a bit. Add in half of chives and eggs. Stir everything for 1 to 2 minutes. Put the cooked eggs over the portobello and sprinkle with remaining

chives. Serve with cherry tomatoes. You can
also eat it with half cup braised spinach.

Lunch: No Fuss Chicken Salad

Fat   : 41 grams
Protein   : 42.7 grams
Net Carbs   : 3.1 grams
Calories   : 560

150 grams cooked chicken thighs, shredded
or chopped

2 hard-boiled pastured eggs, sliced

100 grams lettuce, coarsely shredded

1 tablespoons mayonnaise

Spring onion, coarsely chopped

Salt to taste

Combine all ingredients in a bowl and toss
well to blend flavors. Serve and enjoy.

Dinner: Chops and Asparagus

(See Day 2 for macronutrient details and
recipe)

Dessert: Blueberry and Lemon Cake in a Mug

This recipe makes 5 mugs, and each serving has the following nutrition information:

Fat	: 21 grams
Protein	: 7.2 grams
Net Carbs	: 5.57 grams
Calories	: 188

1/2 cup wild berries, frozen

1/2 cup coconut milk

1/4 cup coconut oil

4 large eggs

1 teaspoon baking soda

1/4 cup Swerve

1/2 cup coconut flour

1 teaspoon coconut flour

1/4 teaspoon Stevia extract

1/2 teaspoon lemon extract

Lemon zest

1/8 teaspoon salt

Get a medium bowl and whisk together baking soda, Swerve, half cup coconut flour, salt, and lemon zest. Add in Stevia, coconut milk, coconut oil, and lemon extract. Get a small bowl and add in 1 teaspoon coconut flour and berries. Toss well to coat evenly. Add berries to batter and combine well. Pour each mug with equal amount of batter. Microwave each mug on high for 1 minute or more. Enjoy your dessert.

Day 7

Breakfast: Sausage and Bell Pepper with Cheese

Fat	: 45 grams
Protein	: 23 grams
Net Carbs	: 9 grams
Calories	: 533

1 ounce sugar-free breakfast sausage, cooked

1 ounce pepper jack cheese, sliced

1 bell pepper

1 tablespoon olive oil

Roast bell pepper in olive oil and put in a plate. Add the cooked sausage and cheese slices. Serve and enjoy.

Lunch: Taco Salad

(See Day 4 for macronutrient details and recipe)

Dinner: Baked Salmon and Faux-tatoes

Fat	: 53 grams
Protein	: 38 grams
Net Carbs	: 6 grams
Calories	: 653

4 ounces Atlantic salmon fillet

1.5 ounces cheddar cheese, grated

1 tablespoon scallions, chopped

1 strip cooked bacon, chopped

2 tablespoons sour cream

1 1/2 tablespoons butter

3/4 cup cauliflower, steamed and mashed

Preheat oven to 350°F. Combine cauliflower, butter, sour cream, bacon, scallions, and cheese in a bowl. Mix well and set aside. Put salmon on a baking dish and bake until browned. Serve salmon with mashed cauliflower.

Dessert: Any Left-Over Dessert from Previous Recipes

If you have left-over desserts, you can consume them but keep you macronutrient requirements in mind.

You can make adjustments to suit your macronutrient requirements. You can use different greens for your green salad each time you prepare it.

You can also prepare 30 grams of pecans, almonds, walnuts, or macadamia nuts for your snack. You can check the list of foods that you are allowed to eat to see what you can grab on the go.

Chapter 4
Managing Yourself and Your Diet

You have your weight loss goal, you know the importance of minimizing your carb consumption, and you have a list of food that you are allowed and not allowed to eat. You should have an idea on how to plan your meal. You still have four more steps to go and you have already passed the most crucial moments in transforming yourself with the help of the ketogenic diet. Keep in mind that you must have realistic time constraints.

Proper Monitoring and Management

Understand that it is best to have gradual transition especially if you are used to eating high-carbs diet. To see a new you, it is important that you properly follow the steps that this book tells you.

After setting the weight that you want to obtain, you must start minimizing your carbs. You can try cutting your usual carb intake first before you start the actual keto diet. You can also choose to start right away but you need to make sure that you will be able to keep up. You can't simply start and stop when you feel like you can't part with your carbs just yet. When you start your keto diet, see to it that you will be able to stick to it no matter what.

You can begin following the sample 7-day meal plan and I suggest looking for other keto recipes that you can use based on your current macronutrients intake. The keto diet calculator is a friend that you can depend on.

It is best to monitor your progress each week. Break your main goal into smaller ones that you can accomplish weekly and make sure to come up with something flexible and reasonable. Understand that you may not see the expected result within that week and you need to make some adjustments. Take note that you only need to check your weight once per week (on the same day each week, as much as possible).

You may need to change some ingredients to help you achieve your target weight for the week. You also need to incorporate physical activities and exercises that can help you tone your body and bring your weight down.

You need to check your macronutrient requirement each month. It will definitely change because your weight and activities also change. If you notice, the keto diet calculator also considers how active you are or your lack of physical activity. It definitely affects your macronutrient requirements to a great degree. Make a careful assessment of everything and provide accurate information so the keto diet calculator can give the most accurate macronutrient estimates.

Measuring your ketone bodies can also help you manage your diet and monitor your progress. You will learn more about the different ways to measure ketone bodies in Chapter 7.

Step 4 to a New You – Move your Body: Exercises and Physical Activities

There are people who thought that exercising while following a ketogenic diet may not bring the expected result or may not yield favorable outcome at all. This idea probably sprung from the fact that keto diet has less carbs and won't be enough to provide the needed amount of fuel that your body needs. Don't forget that fats can also supply the energy that your body needs. In fact, you need to exercise even if you are following a keto diet.

The Different Types of Exercise

Exercise provides many health benefits and you should do it regularly. It strengthens your bones, helps build muscle, and good for the heart. However, you may need to make some adjustments in your nutritional requirements whenever you exercise.

The different types are:

1. Stability

You can have balance and core training as part of your stability exercise. The different trainings improve balance, support alignment, and give you better control of your movement.

2. Flexibility

You can do some stretching and yoga for your flexibility exercise. Flexibility exercises can help increase your range of motion and support soft-tissue as well as help you stretch out your muscle. Enhancing your flexibility can help a lot in preventing injuries due to shortening of muscles.

3. Anaerobic

High intensity interval training (HIIT) and weight lifting can help a lot when doing anaerobic exercise, which provides high intensity carb burning. When doing anaerobic exercise, your primary source of fuel is carbohydrates and that means fat won't be able to provide the needed amount of energy that this type of workout utilizes. It is best to consume more carbohydrates when you choose to do anaerobic exercise.

4. Aerobic

Cardio training is a form of aerobic exercise and it provides low intensity fat burning. A cardio exercise usually lasts more than three minutes. A keto dieter will definitely gain a lot of benefits from this type of exercise.

Adaptation

The intensity of your workout really matters when you are in ketosis. Remember that:

- High-intensity anaerobic exercise has carbohydrates as its primary source of energy.

- Low-intensity aerobic exercise relies on fat as its main energy source.

The good news is that your exercise performance value can greatly increase as your body adapts to the keto diet. It usually takes two to three weeks before your body can get used to relying on fat for fuel. Because your body can't get enough carbohydrates to burn, it will naturally use fat instead.

When you remain on a low-carb and high-fat diet for a long time, your body goes through keto-adaptation. Your body becomes more efficient at burning fat and utilizing ketones as time goes by. The adaptation plays a significant role during exercise.

Even a 30-minute walk everyday can help burn fat and boost your energy level. If you have a tedious task to perform, it is best to consume more fats to power you up when you need an extra energy boost. It is wise to keep your body moving instead of staying put. You can increase your ketone levels during a restricted carb diet if you engage in physical activities.

Chapter 5
Increase Healthy Fats

There are different high quality fats that you can include in your meal to get the most benefits from your keto diet. Studies proved that fats and protein are the most sating nutrients, while the least sating are food rich in carbohydrates. Fat can give a steady supply of energy and you don't need to worry about your insulin because its level won't get affected. You won't experience cravings and mood or energy swings.

Groups of Healthy Fats

1. Saturated Fats (SFAs)

Actual studies proved that there was no significant evidence that saturated fat can increase risk of heart disease, contrary to popular belief. In fact, saturated fats can increase LDL (low density lipoprotein), which is also used to produce hormones like cortisol and testosterone.

There are different sizes of LDL: very small, small, intermediate, and large. Small and very small LDLs are small enough to penetrate arterial wall and cause premature coronary artery disease. On the other hand, large and intermediate LDLs are not linked to elevated heart disease and can bring a lot of benefits to the body. High saturated fat consumption can increase the concentration of large LDLs and lowers the existence of small and very small LDLs according to a study.

Saturated fats can increase concentrations of HDL (high density lipoprotein), which can get bad cholesterol out of your body and hinders build up in the arteries.

Good sources of saturated fats are clarified butter or ghee, coconut oil, duck fat, tallow, lard, butter, goose fat, cocoa butter, palm oil, and chicken fat.

2. Polyunsaturated Fatty Acids (PUFAs)

It is important to remember that PUFAs should not be heated or used for cooking. They can bring a lot of benefits when consumed cold. PUFAs form free radicals when heated. Free radicals are harmful compounds and they can elevate risk of cancer and heart disease to a new height.

There are processed PUFAs (which you need to avoid) and healthy PUFAs from natural sources. PUFAs are rich in omega 3s and omega 6s that can bring a lot of advantages to the body but they should remain balanced in order to get the most benefits. The ideal ratio should be 1:1. However, most Western diets have 1:30 ratio where omega 6 exceeds omega 3 by a huge margin. When you plan to include PUFAs in your keto diet, try to aim for 1:1 ratio.

Good sources of PUFA include omega 3s from seafood and fatty fish, flaxseed oil, extra virgin oil, avocado oil, and nut oils.

3. Monounsaturated Fatty Acids (MUFAs)

For many years, MUFAs have been regarded as healthy fats. There are various studies that linked them to better insulin resistance and good cholesterol. The following are the health benefits of monounsaturated fats on ketosis:

- Lower insulin resistance

- Occurrence of flatter tummy

- Lower heart disease risk

- More HDL

- Prevent hypertension or high blood pressure

Good sources of MUFAs are extra virgin olive oil, macadamia nut oil, goose fat, lard, bacon fat, and avocado oil.

4. Natural Trans Fats

Most trans fats are harmful and unhealthy because they are processed, but natural trans fats are different. The harmful trans fats went through a process called hydrogenation, which has the ability to keep polyunsaturated oils from becoming rancid (you already know that PUFAs must not be heated). Hydrogenated fats are commonly used in fast foods, commercially baked goodies, margarine, and processed foods (canned goods and others).

Natural trans fats did not go through hydrogenation and no nutrient was compromised. You can be certain that you will get nothing but natural goodness of the beneficial type of trans fats.

Good sources of trans fats include dairy fats like yogurt and butter, products from grass-fed animal.

5. MCTs

Adding MCT oil into your diet can help a lot in managing your weight as it balances hormones that can suppress your hunger, increases metabolism, and supports ketosis. MCTs can greatly improve athletic performance.

MCTs are capable of combating harmful parasites, fungi, viruses, and bacteria. Moreover, they also have antioxidant properties. Medium-chain fatty acids can help you absorb the different foods' fat-soluble nutrients.

Good sources of MCTs include coconut oil, palm oil, and MCT oils.

Consuming large amount of fats can help increase ketone production. Functional benefits of ketones include:

- Beneficial effect on mental performance. A large part of your brain needs energy to perform well and ketones can efficiently provide it while on ketogenic diet.

- Extra energy during workouts. Your body consumes more fuel when you exercise and it is only right to supply it with steady source of energy.

But you still need to maintain the ideal ketone levels, too much of everything can bring more harm than good.

Step 5 to a New You – Add Vigor and Consume Healthy Fats

Each fat burns differently and gives varied amount of energy. There are fats or oils that must not be used for cooking. Here is a list of healthy fats and oils that you can add to your keto diet:

	FAT / OIL	% SFA	% MUFA	% PUFA	*ω-6 : ω-3 Ratio
Goo d for Coo	Red Palm Oil	52	39	10	2 : 1
	Lard	40	45	11	12 : 1

king	Grass-Fed Tallow	47	41	8	1.5 : 1
	Goose Fat	28	57	11	12 : 1
	Ghee	65	32	3	1 : 1
	Duck Fat	33	50	13	12 : 1
	Coconut Oil	87	6	2	2 : 1
	Cocoa Butter	60	33	3	3 : 1
	Chicken Fat	30	45	21	12 : 1
	Butter	65	32	3	1 : 1
Light Cooking Only & Cold Use	Macadamia Oil	16	83	1	2 : 1
	Extra Virgin Olive Oil	14	73	11	11 : 1
	Avocado Oil	11	71	14	12 : 1
Strictly for Cold Use Only	Walnut Oil	9	28	63	7 : 1
	Sesame Oil	15	40	45	45 : 1
	Pumpkin Seed Oil	17	20	63	20 : 1
	Pistachio Oil	15	54	31	31 : 1

Peanut Oil	17	46	32	34 : 1
Hazelnut Oil	10	75	15	15 : 1
Flaxseed Oil	9	18	73	.3 : 1
Fish Oil	20 / 30	27 / 57	15 / 40	1:6 / 1:8
Almond Oil	7	65	28	28 : 1

* ω means omega

Different Ways to Increase your Fat Intake

When you cook your food, make sure to cook with the right kind of fat. The list above can serve as your guide. Not all fats or oils can be used for cooking. Choose the recommended oils or fats for cooking when frying your meat, sautéing your vegetables, or cooking your other dishes that require fat or oil.

Prepare salad using extra virgin olive oil or other oils that are suitable for cold use and/or light cooking.

You can melt some butter or add coconut oil in your tea or coffee for a quick and easy fat boost. You can also try adding some heavy whipping cream.

There are fat bombs dessert recipes in this book that you can prepare. You can eat as many as you want but still be mindful of your ideal macronutrient intake (different people have different macronutrient ratios).

Add as much fat or oil as you need and remember that not all of them can be used for cooking.

Chapter 6
Maintain Adequate Protein Intake

You need protein to have all the essential amino acids that your body needs. You need protein to help you with the proper functioning of organs and tissues in your body.

When following a ketogenic diet, most people tend to add protein to replace a large portion of carbohydrates from their usual diet. More protein is not always good and it can keep you out of ketosis.

A ketogenic diet must have lots of fats, moderate amount of protein, and less carbohydrates.

Step 6 to a New You – Maintain the Right Protein Amount

If you eat too much protein, your body can turn amino acids into glucose for energy. This can spike your insulin and reduce the presence of ketones in your blood. You might even experience keto flu due to unstable ketosis. That's why it's important to follow the macronutrient proportion that the keto diet calculator has recommended.

When measuring your ideal macronutrient intake, you need to consider your gender, weight, height, age, body fat, physical activities, and other important factors. When you use the keto diet calculator, you will get your ideal macronutrient intake and just follow the recommendation.

Remember that the portion that you allot for fats in your diet should be the biggest.

Chapter 7
Test / Measure Ketone Levels

There are different ways to measure ketone levels. People who follow a ketogenic diet usually do regular tests to know their current levels of ketosis and ketones.

The Different Tests

Urine Testing

You can buy urine strips that measure ketone level by color. When you use this method, just follow the manufacturer's guide to determine your ketone level. You simply pee on your urine strip and match the result with the manufacturer's guide.

This is an affordable and quick option if you want to know your ketone level. However, for someone who has been in a keto diet for a long time, the urine test may not be able to give accurate results.

Blood Testing

To do this, you need a lancet pen. You press the pen onto the tip of your finger to draw blood, which must be applied on a test strip that can determine ketone levels using a meter.

This method is quite accurate in testing your ketone level but it can be expensive, especially if you conduct your test frequently. The meter itself is around $40 and each test strip is around $5 to $10.

Breath Testing

You can also use a Ketonix breath meter to test the presence of acetone in your breath and determine the amount.

Once you buy the meter, you can use it as much as you want without the need to spend extra. It is best to use this together with other methods because it is not that reliable.

You need to test your ketone level to make sure that your body remains in ketosis. You can buy the materials you need at online shops as well as Wal-mart, local pharmacy, and similar establishments.

Step 7 to a New You – Measure your Ketones

When monitoring your ketone levels, you need to keep these in mind:

1. Ketone concentrations are lower during daytime and higher at nighttime. If you prefer to measure your ketone level in the morning, make sure to be consistent and always take it during daytime.

2. Expect fluctuations due to everyday changes in hormone levels.

3. The amount of fats in your diet can affect your ketone level. You may need to adjust accordingly or consume foods that contain MCT to help you boost your ketones.

4. Try consuming fat bombs with 80% fat content.

5. When your breath seems to give off a "fruity" smell, drink lots of water and consume food that are rich in electrolytes. Drinking mint tea also helps.

6. Keep your body active or do extensive aerobic exercise, it can help you get into ketosis almost immediately.

You measure your ketones to make sure that you are not going off track. You don't need to measure every day but you need to follow a regular schedule so you can monitor properly.

Chapter 8
Bonus Tip – Intermittent Fasting

Aside from ketogenic diet, intermittent fasting can also help increase your ketone levels. As the name implies, it is a form of fasting where you are also allowed to eat but for a limited time. You also fast when you sleep.

Intermittent fasting has eating period and fasting period. It has no restriction on the type of food that you consume, although it is recommended to eat more organic vegetables and fruits. As you can see, it is more lax than keto diet when it comes to the types of food that you need to consume. However, it strictly prohibits eating during fasting period and you need to prepare foods that can make you feel full longer.

Beauty of Intermittent Fasting

Intermittent fasting can make you lose weight, improve your metabolic health, and fend off disease. It may even be possible for you to live longer when you follow intermittent fasting.

Intermittent fasting requires you to eat and then fast. Believe it or not, people "fast" each day. On normal days, you fast while you are sleeping or working non-stop to finish your work. You fast if you are unable to eat anything for a longer period of time than normal.

There are numerous people who claimed that they felt better and more energetic after fasting for a long time. It is natural to feel extremely hungry on the first few days, but you will be able to adapt as time goes by.

During fasting period, you are not permitted to eat anything but you are allowed to drink water. You can also drink young coconut water, homemade infused water, tea, coffee, and other non-caloric drinks. Prepare fruit infused water if you don't want to drink bland water all the time. Commercial fruit infused water is loaded with sugar, which is unhealthy.

You are allowed to take supplements when fasting and make sure that they don't contain calories. When you fast, your glucose and insulin levels go down, while the level of your growth hormones goes up.

People who want to lose weight turn to intermittent fasting. It is simple to do and can effectively burn fat and restrict caloric intake. It also provides metabolic health benefits. It can help protect your body against numerous diseases, such as Type 2 diabetes, certain cancer, heart disease, and others.

On the practical side, following intermittent fasting can save you some money. Instead of eating three or four meals per day, you only need to eat two. Preparing your meal and cleaning up also become easier than before. You will be fit and healthy. You will also feel light and get a lot of other benefits.

What Happens during Eating and Fasting?

Eating period usually takes 4 to 12 hours. The food you consumed gets digested and absorbed by your body. When you eat, your insulin level rises and it becomes impossible for your body to burn fats. Your body uses glucose as fuel because insulin made it so.

When eating period ends, your body stops processing food, and fasting period begins.

During fasting period, your body has no other option but burn fats because your insulin level is low. Take note that your insulin level won't immediately diminish just because you stopped eating. It usually takes three to five hours for your body to start burning fat and will continue to do so while you are in your fasting period. Ketosis happens as you burn fats.

Different Types of Intermittent Fasting

There are different kinds of intermittent fasting and you can choose the schedule that fits your preference. The different kinds of intermittent fasting are:

1) 12-hour Fast

Your eating period is set for 12 hours and your fasting period is also set for 12 hours. This type of intermittent fasting is best for beginners.

2) 8-hour Window

This type of intermittent fasting requires fasting for 14 to 16 hours every day. You can only eat for 8 to 10 hours and not have anything after that. The best way to accomplish this is to skip breakfast, eat your lunch, eat some snacks, eat your dinner, and then stop eating. When you calculate the time, from lunch to dinner, you have 8 to 10 hours to eat. After you finished eating, your fasting period begins.

3) 20:4 Method

This requires you to fast for 20 hours every day, which means you only have 4 hours eating period. You can eat anytime and anything within your eating period. It is recommended to still choose healthy and fulfilling meals. Choose the ones that can make you feel full for a long time. It is also best to avoid eating sweet things. After 4 hours, you need to fast in the next 20 hours. If you follow this type of intermittent fasting, you can do it once, twice, or thrice a week. As a beginner, it is too soon to do it every day because your body may not be able to cope and your effort will be wasted.

4) 5:2 Plan

This type of intermittent fasting allows you to eat normal, healthy meals for five consecutive days. You are required to restrict your caloric intake for the next two days. A woman should only consume a total of 500 calories per day, while men should eat a total of 600 calories per day.

When you follow this method, you need to have lots of vegetables, good fats, and protein. You can distribute your caloric intake like this:

- 100 calories for breakfast

- 200 calories for lunch

-200 / 300 calories for dinner

You can drink lots of liquids, especially water, to help you feel full. It is important to avoid drinking sugary beverages.

There are other types of intermittent fasting but the listed types are enough to give you an idea about what it can do to your body.

Conclusion

Thank you again for downloading this book!

I hope this book has provided you with enough information about the ketogenic diet, ketones, ketosis, and how the keto diet can help you discover a new you.

To wrap things up:

1. You must be clear on your weight loss goal before you start your keto diet. It is highly recommended to have an accountability partner that can help you monitor your progress and see to it that you don't deviate from your goal.

2. Minimize your carb consumption to attain a less bumpy transition. Don't expect it to be smooth, especially if you are used to eating the usual Western diet. You can introduce coconut oil and MCT oil in your diet for extra fats.

3. Plan your keto meal and include snacks on the go during those days when you don't have time to prepare.

4. Make sure to exercise regularly and try to increase your physical activity. Even a walk around the park can help you tone your body and burn some fats.

5. Increase your fat intake and see the difference in your vitality. Keep in mind that there are fats or oils that must not be heated.

6. Make sure to maintain the right amount of protein to prevent falling out of ketosis or having keto flu.

7. Monitor and measure your ketone bodies to track your progress and make sure that you are in ketosis.

I hope that the bonus chapter about intermittent fasting has provided additional information that you can use to improve yourself even better.

If you enjoyed this book, please take the time to share your thoughts and post a review on Amazon. It'd be greatly appreciated!

Thank you and good luck!

www.ingramcontent.com/pod-product-compliance
Lightning Source LLC
Chambersburg PA
CBHW060748260726
48660CB00002B/536